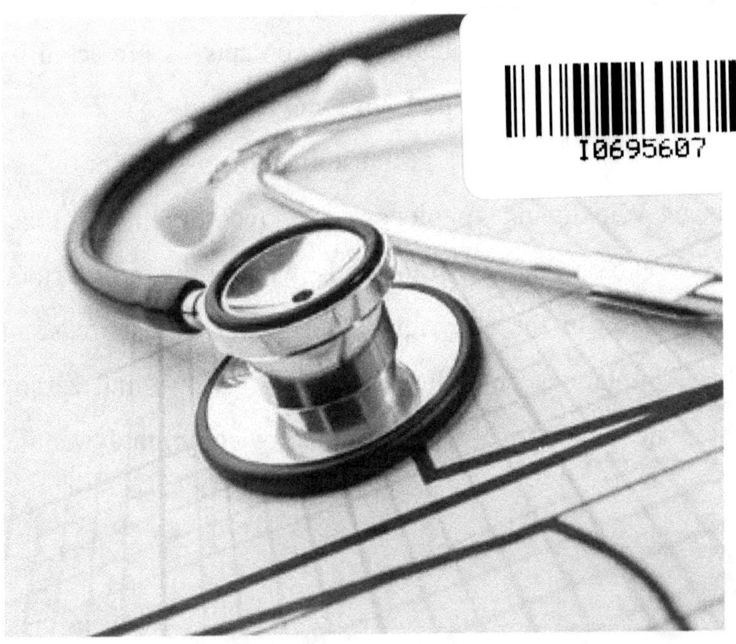

The Cardiologist's Secrets:

Your Ultimate Guide to Preventing and Controlling Hypertension

DR. JOHN TAYLOR

TABLE OF CONTENT

Overview of Hypertension

One summer afternoon, madam, Caroline, a 43-year-old previously diagnosed hypertensive, walked into the cardiologist's office I was working with in a teaching hospital. She reported that day on account of sudden onset of headaches, dizziness, palpitations, insomnia, easy tiredness, and dyspnea lying supine.

Though she was put on three blood pressure medications, she reported to the office with a blood pressure of 186/108mmHg and a heart rate of 115 beats per minute.

Her social history revealed that she grew up near the sea where she consumed a lot of seafood including high salt. She worked in a reputable bank as a manager. Her work schedule is very tight; she mostly drives to work and barely closes early. The earliest she takes supper is 6 pm to 7 pm. Her mother passed away some years ago on account of sudden cardiac arrest, and her brother was diagnosed with hypertension some three years after her diagnosis.

On examination, she looked anxious and agitated. Her laboratory results revealed a deranged thyroid function test. The cardiologist reviewed her medication and counseled her. She reported back to the hospital once weekly, twice monthly, and finally monthly. Within the next three months, she had her blood pressure well controlled at 124/88mmHg and, a heart rate of 82 beats per minute. More so, she was not exhibiting any signs or symptoms of cardiac, thyroid, or renal impairment.

Over my five years of attachment with the cardiologist, we prevented, controlled, and treated many patients with impending organ failure due to high blood pressure. This book is written to help you and all those who are genetically exposed to high blood pressure, those who are socially, occupationally, and environmentally exposed, those who have blood pressure, and those with complications of blood pressure to take control of their heart health and live a health life.

In the tapestry of our lives, the heartbeat is the rhythm that orchestrates our existence. Yet, lurking in the shadows is a silent intruder, hypertension, threatening to disrupt this harmonious melody. The importance of hypertension prevention cannot be overstated, for it is not merely a matter of safeguarding against a single condition but a holistic commitment to nurturing heart health and preserving the symphony of our well-being.

This handbook is a roadmap, a companion on your journey to well-being. As we delve into the following pages, let's unravel the mysteries of hypertension, explore the pathways to prevention, and embrace the collective strength of our community to cultivate heart health.

Heart Health Facts

Guardian of Vital Organs: The heart is at the forefront of the battle against hypertension. By preventing high blood pressure, you shield vital organs such as the heart, brain, and kidneys from the potential ravages of sustained pressure.

Economic and Social Empowerment: The economic and social implications of hypertension are profound. Prevention translates into a healthier workforce, reduced healthcare costs, and an empowered community capable of actively contributing to the fabric of society

Break the Generational Cycle: Hypertension often weaves a silent thread through families, passing from one generation to the next. Prevention is not only a gift to ourselves but a legacy bestowed upon our children and generations to come.

Breaking the cycle of hypertension ensures a lineage endowed with the knowledge and tools to lead heart-healthy lives.

Holistic Well-Being: Hypertension prevention is a commitment to holistic well-being. It encompasses the delicate balance between mind, body, and spirit. By embracing preventive measures, we foster mental resilience, emotional equilibrium, and a sense of interconnectedness that transcends the boundaries of our physical health.

Empowerment Through Knowledge: Knowledge is the compass guiding us on the path to prevention. By understanding the factors contributing to hypertension and the proactive steps to mitigate its risks, we empower ourselves with the tools needed to make informed choices.

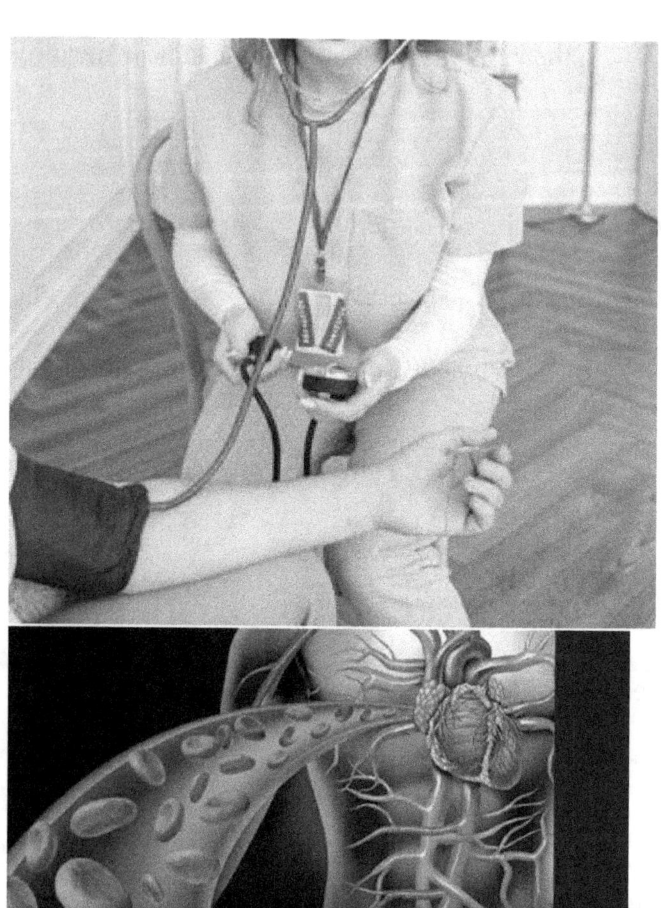

CHAPTER ONE

Definition of Hypertension

Blood Pressure also called hypertension at its core, is the force of blood against the walls of the blood vessels-arteries. When this force exceeds normal levels, it sets the stage for potential health complications. There is usually a normal pressure in the arteries which must be maintained at all times. This force should not go lower or higher than the normal. Whilst both pose a danger to human health, high blood pressure is the most common. This book on blood pressure intends to help you prevent high blood pressure. Blood pressure is measured using two values – systolic pressure, representing the force when the heart beats, and diastolic pressure, reflecting the force when the heart is at rest or relaxing. The unit of measurement is millimeters of mercury (mmHg).

While a blood pressure reading of 120/80 mmHg is considered normal, hypertension manifests when readings consistently rise above this threshold. Hypertension is classified depending on recorded values or based on the causes. The American Heart Association classifies blood pressure into several categories based on the recording of the sphygmomanometer:

Normal: 100-120/60-80 mmHg

Elevated: 120-129/<80 mmHg

Stage 1 Hypertension/Pre-hypertension:

130-139/80-89 mmHg

Stage 2 Hypertension: 140-180 /90-120mmHg

Hypertensive Crisis: Higher than >180/>120 mmHg

Hypertension can also be classified as:

Essential/primary hypertension: this refers to blood pressure without any underlying medical conditions. Mostly this is caused by the three main factors including diet, exercise, and stress.

Nonessential hypertension/secondary hypertension: refers to elevated blood pressure with a specific underlying cause or identifiable contributing factor. Unlike essential hypertension, which is primarily influenced by genetic and lifestyle factors, nonessential hypertension is linked to a variety of medical conditions or external influences. Some of these causes include:

Renal Causes: renal artery stenosis, Polycystic kidney disease, and, Chronic kidney disease

Endocrine Causes: primary hyperaldosteronism, Cushing's syndrome, hyperthyroidism, or hypothyroidism

Sleep Apnea: obstructive sleep apnea has been linked to hypertension, potentially due to intermittent hypoxia and increased sympathetic activity.

Epidemiology of Hypertension

The prevalence of hypertension is a global health concern, affecting a substantial portion of the population and contributing significantly to disease and death.

Hypertension is a pervasive health issue worldwide, impacting individuals across diverse demographics. Hypertension tends to increase with age, with a higher prevalence observed in older populations. In certain age groups, men may have a higher prevalence of hypertension than women, while women may experience an increased risk after menopause.

Urbanization is often associated with an increased prevalence of hypertension due to lifestyle changes, including poor dietary habits, stress, sedentary lifestyle, and reduced physical activity.

CHAPTER TWO

Hypertension Pathway

Essential hypertension has a multifaceted and intricate etiology. The kidney is both the target and a contributing organ in hypertensive processes and the illness is caused by a variety of mechanisms involving independent or dependent pathways as well as the interplay of several organ systems.

Genetics, obesity, elevated dietary salt intake, and the activation of neurohormonal systems including the renin-angiotensin-aldosterone system and sympathetic nervous system are some of the key factors that contribute to the pathophysiology of hypertension.

Systemic blood pressure (BP) increase that persists is known as arterial hypertension. The sum of cardiac output and total peripheral vascular resistance is known as blood pressure. Both short-term and long-term blood pressure regulation for sufficient tissue perfusion is influenced by several factors, which include heart output and blood volume in circulation, vascular reactivity, elasticity, and caliber, stimulation of neurons

Essential hypertension evolves from sporadic to chronic hypertension over its natural history. Persistent hypertension evolves into complex hypertension during a protracted, consistent, asymptomatic period during which there is obvious target organ damage to the heart, kidneys, retina, aorta, and minor arteries as well as the central nervous system.

Essential hypertension progresses as follows: prehypertension in people ages 10 to 30 (due to an increase in cardiac output); early hypertension in people ages 20 to 40 (due to a prominent increase in peripheral resistance);

established hypertension in people ages 30 to 50; and complicated hypertension in people ages 40 to 60.

During my years of clinical work with a cardiologist, he used to tell his clients that hypertension is 3+1+1. The 3 represents three things we can modify to prevent high blood pressure. These are diet or nutrition, exercise, and stress. The first "1" represents chronic medical conditions that lead to hypertension and the last "1" represents genetic predisposition. These factors are explained further below.

Diet and nutrition

The food we consume is a powerful determinant of our cardiovascular health. High sodium intake, commonly found in processed foods, can elevate blood pressure. Conversely, diets rich in potassium, calcium, and magnesium have been associated with lower blood pressure levels. The Dietary

Approaches to Stop Hypertension (DASH) diet is a notable example, emphasizing fruits, vegetables, whole grains, and lean proteins.

Exercise

A sedentary lifestyle is a known contributor to hypertension. Exercise has been shown to enhance endothelial function, which plays a crucial role in regulating blood vessel tone. Exercise has been linked to a reduction in sympathetic nervous system activity. Regular exercise also helps in weight management, maintaining a healthy weight, and preventing obesity. It also improves insulin sensitivity, positively impacting blood pressure regulation. Insulin resistance is associated with hypertension, and regular physical activity helps mitigate this risk. These reductions can contribute to lower blood pressure in individuals with hypertension

Regular physical activity helps maintain a healthy weight and promotes cardiovascular fitness, contributing to the overall well-being of our circulatory system.

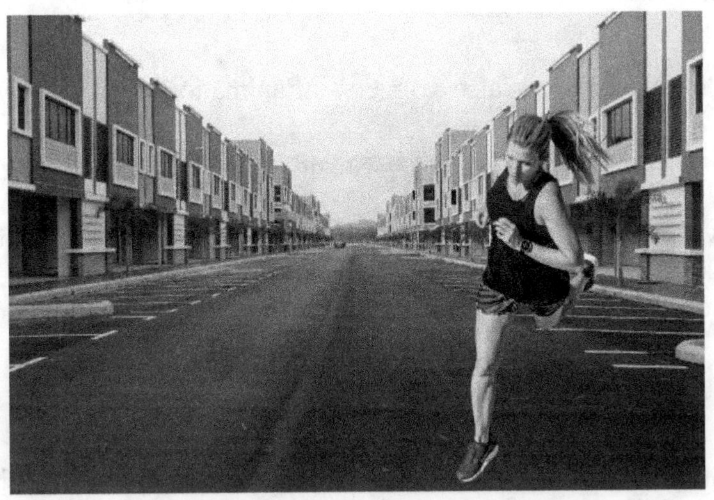

A lady Exercising for Physical Fitness

Stress

The demands of modern life often subject us to chronic stress, impacting our blood pressure. Stress triggers a cascade of physiological responses in the body, including the release of stress hormones like cortisol and adrenaline. These hormones, designed to prepare the body for a "fight or flight" response, can lead to a temporary increase in blood pressure.

Prolonged stress also triggers inflammation in the body, including the vascular system. Inflammation is associated with arterial stiffness and damage, contributing to the development and progression of pressure in the blood vessels.

Stress often accompanies unhealthy lifestyle choices, such as poor dietary habits, lack of exercise, and disrupted sleep patterns. These factors, when combined with stress, create a synergistic effect, exacerbating the risk of developing hypertension. Individuals under chronic stress may be more prone to engaging in behaviors that are detrimental to their cardiovascular health.

However, chronic exposure to stress can result in sustained elevated blood pressure levels.

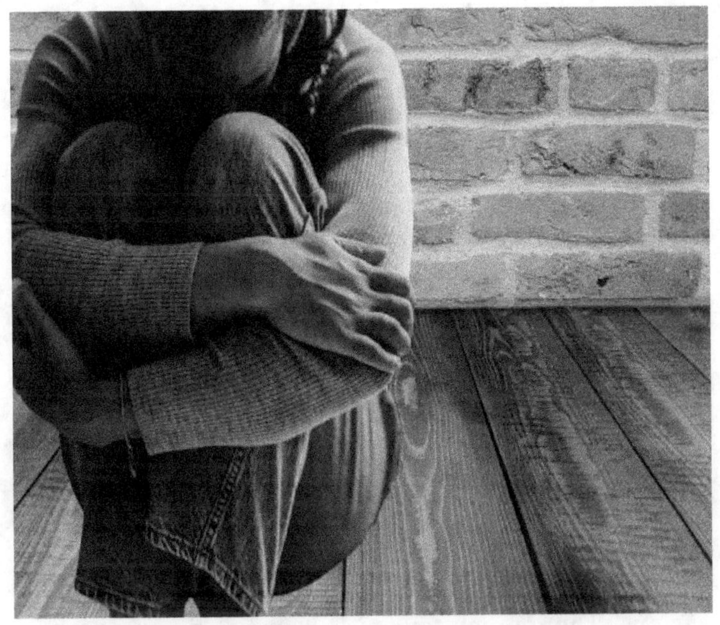

Chronic stress at an early age predisposes one to hypertension

Genetic Factors

While genetics play a role in hypertension, it is crucial to understand that family history does not dictate destiny. If hypertension runs in your family, the likelihood of developing hypertension is high.

As we age, the risk of hypertension tends to increase. Additionally, men are generally at a higher risk until the age of 64, after which the risk becomes comparable between genders. Understanding the age and gender dynamics of hypertension allows for targeted preventive strategies at different life stages.

By recognizing the interconnected influences shaping our blood pressure, we gain the power to make informed decisions. The journey toward hypertension prevention is a personalized one, and understanding these factors equips us with the tools to navigate it successfully. As we embark on this exploration, let us bear in mind that each choice we make today is a step towards a heart-healthy tomorrow.

Underlying chronic medical conditions

Individuals grappling with chronic medical conditions often experience heightened stress. The daily challenges, routine medications, uncertainties, and lifestyle adjustments associated with conditions such as diabetes, chronic kidney disease, and autoimmune disorders can contribute to an elevated stress response. Recognizing these stressors and proper management of chronic medical conditions is fundamental to addressing their impact on blood pressure.

Individuals living with chronic pain or discomfort due to conditions such as arthritis or migraines often contend with heightened stress levels. Persistent pain can trigger the body's stress response, leading to increased blood pressure. Conditions like sleep apnea or insomnia not only disrupt sleep patterns but also contribute to increased stress. Poor sleep quality activates stress hormones and negatively impacts blood pressure regulation. Mental health conditions, including anxiety and depression, are intricately linked with stress and hypertension.

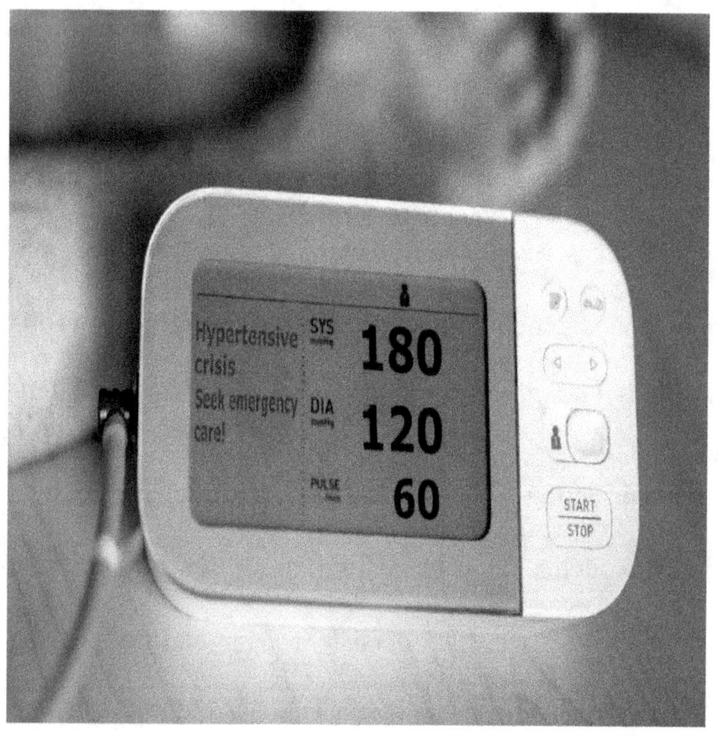

Hypertensive Crises

CHAPTER THREE

How to Recognize Hypertension

In all my years of clinical work, I have realized that more than half of patients get surprised when they are told of having high blood pressure. One of the hallmark characteristics of hypertension is its silent progression. In many cases, individuals may be unaware of elevated blood pressure levels until complications arise or are detected through routine monitoring.

Routine blood pressure monitoring, therefore, becomes a vital tool for early detection of impending heart diseases. Regular blood pressure checking is the ultimate means of detecting high blood pressure in humans because the condition does not give bodily signals of ill health in the elevated and prehypertension stages until complications set in. The clinical manifestations of hypertensive crises are therefore mostly dependent on the organ that is affected.

Patients exhibit cardiac failure symptoms if the heart is affected or renal symptoms if the kidney gets affected. Some patients present at the physician's office with symptoms of multisystem dysfunction.

Symptoms of hypertension

Elevated Blood Pressure Readings: The first sign of hypertension is consistently elevated blood pressure readings above the normal. It is important to note that an individual can have transient elevated blood pressure during times of acute pain, panic, or emotional instability. Improper blood pressure monitoring techniques can also lead to low or high blood pressure recordings. Regular proper monitoring of blood pressure is therefore crucial for identifying hypertension. Elevated readings, especially consistently high systolic (top number) and diastolic (bottom number) values, may indicate hypertension. Consistent blood pressure readings above 130/80 mm Hg warrant attention and further assessment.

Headaches: Headaches are a common complaint that is associated with almost every condition. Hypertension crises are sometimes associated with headaches. Persistent, throbbing headaches, especially at the back of the head and during the morning, may warrant assessment for high blood pressure and its risk factors.

Dizziness and Lightheadedness: Episodes of dizziness or lightheadedness, particularly when standing up, may be indicative of blood pressure fluctuations. Monitoring for these symptoms can offer early clues to potential hypertension.

Vision Changes: Hypertension can impact the small blood vessels in vital organs such as the eyes, leading to changes in vision. Blurred or distorted vision and, in severe cases, increased ocular pressure or vision loss may be signs of uncontrolled hypertension.

Chest Pain and Shortness of Breath: In cases where hypertension has led to complications such as heart disease, individuals may experience chest pain or discomfort and shortness of breath. These symptoms necessitate immediate medical attention.

Fatigue and Difficulty Sleeping: Chronic fatigue and difficulty sleeping can be linked to hypertension. The increased strain on the cardiovascular system may disrupt sleep patterns and contribute to overall fatigue.

Swollen feet: swelling in the legs, ankles, or feet can be a sign of hypertension, indicating that the heart is struggling to pump blood efficiently.

CHAPTER FOUR

Blood Pressure Monitoring Techniques

Regular blood pressure monitoring is a crucial aspect of hypertension prevention, offering valuable insights into cardiovascular health. Understanding how to measure and interpret blood pressure readings empowers individuals to take proactive steps toward maintaining optimal heart health.

Empowering Self-Care: Home blood pressure monitoring provides individuals with the ability to track their blood pressure in familiar and relaxed settings. This empowerment fosters a sense of personal responsibility and aids in the early detection of potential issues.

Comprehensive Picture: Blood pressure differs slightly among people and also fluctuates throughout the day. Many factors can affect blood pressure readings during the day. Systolic blood pressure may increase during times of stress or emotional instability. Incorporating home monitoring into a hypertension prevention plan offers a more comprehensive picture of blood pressure trends within a period. Regular monitoring at different times of the day under varying conditions allows individuals and their healthcare providers to identify patterns, assess the effectiveness of lifestyle changes, and make informed decisions about their health.

Automatic vs. Manual Monitors: Automatic blood pressure monitors are user-friendly and often preferred for at-home use. Manual monitors, while accurate, may require more skill in operation. Healthcare professionals prefer manual blood pressure monitors to automatic machines to due their accuracy. Most people who do blood pressure monitoring at home need an automatic monitoring machine instead manual monitor.

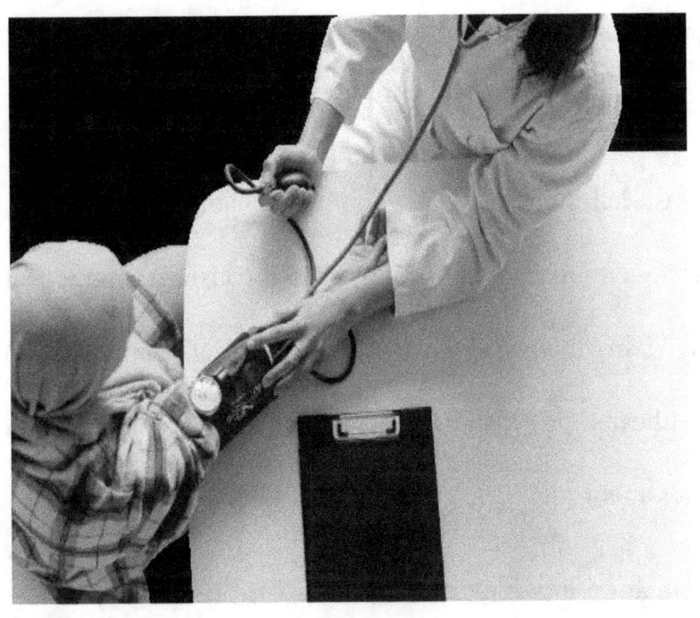

Manual Blood Pressure Monitoring

Taking measurements: Ensuring the correct cuff size is crucial for accurate readings. Using an improperly sized cuff can result in misleading blood pressure measurements. Before blood pressure measurement, one needs to rest for at least thirty minutes and feel relaxed. Maintaining a correct posture during blood pressure measurement is paramount. It is appropriate to sit upright with a blood pressure machine at heart level.

Consistency is Key: To obtain reliable readings, it is essential to measure blood pressure at consistent times of the day. This helps identify any fluctuations and provides healthcare professionals with valuable information for assessment.

Maintain a log of these blood pressure readings, including the date and time. This chart serves as a valuable tool during medical appointments and enables healthcare providers to make informed decisions about hypertension prevention strategies.

Understanding Blood Pressure Readings

Systolic and Diastolic Values: Blood pressure readings consist of two values - systolic (pressure during heartbeats) and diastolic (pressure between heartbeats). Understanding the significance of both values provides a comprehensive understanding of cardiovascular health

Blood pressure readings are categorized into different ranges. For instance:

Normal: 100-120/60-80 mmHg

Elevated: 120-129/<80 mmHg

Stage 1 Hypertension/Pre-hypertension:

130-139/80-89 mmHg

Stage 2 Hypertension: 140-180 /90-120mmHg

Hypertensive Crisis: Higher than >180/>120 mmHg

In conclusion, understanding these values is crucial for early initiation of intervention. Monitoring blood pressure severally to understand one's baseline readings is essential in making a definite diagnosis of hypertension.

It is there important for everyone to regularly monitor blood pressure at home since the disease is asymptomatic and can lead to sudden death. While hypertension may be asymptomatic in its early stages, being attuned to subtle cues and engaging in regular blood pressure monitoring is the first line of defense in preventing its progression.

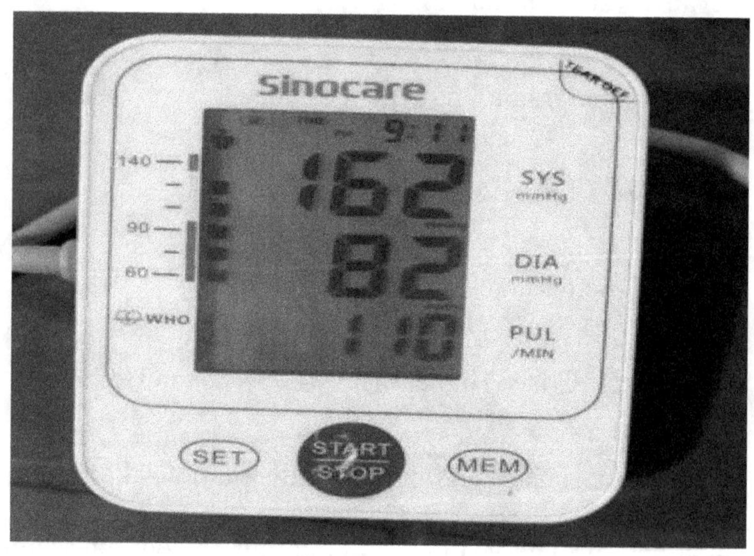

CHAPTER FIVE

Strategies to Prevent Hypertension

Understanding the impact of lifestyle choices is pivotal in the quest for hypertension prevention. This section explains key lifestyle risk factors that can contribute to elevated blood pressure and offers insights into how to modify these factors since this is the cornerstone of your journey toward a heart-healthy lifestyle. The 3 modifiable lifestyle factors include diet, exercise, and stress.

Diet and Nutrition

DASH Diet Technique for Hypertension Prevention

DASH is an acronym for **Dietary Approaches to Stop Hypertension**. Diet plays a pivotal role in hypertension prevention, and one dietary approach that has demonstrated remarkable effectiveness is the DASH diet. Developed by the National Heart, Lung, and Blood Institute, the DASH diet is not just a temporary fix but a sustainable lifestyle approach designed to lower blood pressure and promote overall cardiovascular health. Let's explore the key principles and techniques of the DASH diet for hypertension prevention and management.

Understanding the DASH Diet

The DASH diet is characterized by a balanced and heart-healthy approach to eating. It emphasizes nutrient-rich, whole foods while reducing sodium intake. The core components include:

Fruits and Vegetables: Aim to include a variety of colorful fruits and vegetables in your daily meals. These foods are rich in potassium, which helps balance sodium levels and regulate blood pressure. Additionally, they are rich in vitamins, minerals, and antioxidants which help reduce inflammation and oxidative stress. The fiber in fruits and vegetables also aids in digestion and weight management which help support overall cardiovascular health.

Whole Grains: Show preferences for whole grains over refined foods. Consume whole grains such as quinoa, brown rice, and whole wheat bread instead of refined grains. Whole grains contain a good amount of fiber and some other essential nutrients which promote heart health.

Lean Proteins: opt for lean protein sources, including fish, beans, nuts, and seeds. These proteins contribute to overall health without the saturated fats in other protein sources.

Dairy or Dairy Alternatives: Include low-fat or fat-free dairy products or dairy alternatives to ensure an adequate intake of calcium and vitamin D.

Nuts, Seeds, and Legumes: Incorporate these into your diet for added nutrients, healthy fats, and protein.

Limit Saturated and Trans Fats: Reduce the intake of saturated and trans fats, commonly found in processed and fried foods, to support heart health.

The DASH diet places a strong emphasis on reducing sodium, a key contributor to hypertension.

Techniques to minimize sodium intake

Reading Food Labels: When buying packaged foods, pay attention to the amount of sodium in the food. Wherever possible, go for alternates that are low in or free of salt.

Use Herbs and Spices: Flavor meals with herbs, spices, and other seasonings instead of salt. In doing so, the flavor of the food is improved without compromising heart health.

Cooking at Home: Home-cooked meals allow better control over ingredients, reducing the reliance on high-sodium restaurants or processed foods.

Reduction of sodium consumption: High sodium consumption is a prominent contributor to hypertension. Processed foods, restaurant meals, and pre-packaged snacks often harbor hidden sodium. Understanding food labels and opting for fresh, whole foods can significantly reduce sodium intake.

Potassium-rich foods: A potassium deficiency can exacerbate hypertension. Embracing a diet rich in fruits, vegetables, and potassium-containing foods, such as bananas, oranges, and leafy greens, can help maintain a healthy balance.

Hydration: Adequate hydration is crucial. Choose water over sugary beverages, and limit alcohol intake.

Portion Control and Balanced Meals: Portion control refers to managing the amount of food you eat at a meal or snack to ensure you are consuming an appropriate serving size. It involves being mindful of how much you are consuming relative to recommended serving sizes and your own nutritional needs. Maintaining a healthy weight is essential for hypertension prevention. The DASH diet encourages portion control and the creation of balanced meals to ensure a diverse and nutritious intake.

Techniques to achieve portion control

1. **Use smaller plates:** Opting for smaller dishware during meals naturally helps to limit the quantity of food to consume

2. **Measure the serving size:** use measuring cups, spoons, or a food scale to accurately portion out the food to be eaten.

3. **Be familiar with portion sizes: Be mindful of** the recommended portion sizes for different food groups and try to stick to them.

4. **Fill half of your plate with fruits and vegetables:** fill about half of your plate with fruits and vegetables to help control overall calorie intake while ensuring you get essential nutrients

5. **Practice the plate method:** divide your plate into sections for protein, grains, and vegetables with vegetables taking up the largest portion

6. **Eat slowly and listen to body hunger and fullness cues:** eat slowly and focus on the taste, texture, and experience of eating. This helps your body to register feelings of fullness, helping to prevent overeating. It also helps to stop eating when satisfied rather than when the plate is empty.

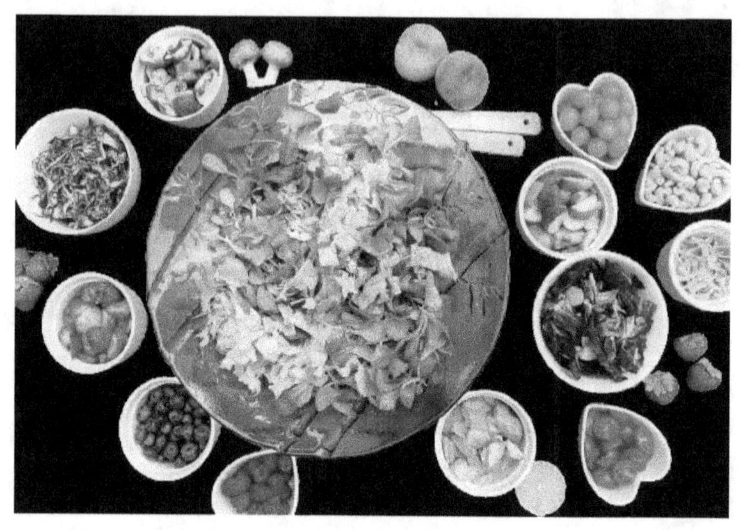

Physical Activity

A lack of physical activity can contribute to weight gain and elevate blood pressure. Incorporating regular aerobic exercise, such as brisk walking or cycling, as well as strength training, not only aids in weight management but also supports cardiovascular health.

Moderation and Consistency: Engaging in moderate-intensity exercise most days of the week is beneficial. For every week, strive for at least 150 minutes of moderate-intensity or 75 minutes of vigorous-intensity exercise, combined with two or more days of muscle-strengthening exercise.

Age-Specific Exercise Guidelines for Hypertension Prevention

Exercise is a cornerstone of hypertension prevention, contributing not only to physical well-being but also to promoting cardiovascular health. Many patients asked their healthcare practitioners what exercise is appropriate for them and for how long they should do it.

Therefore, tailoring an exercise schedule to age-specific needs ensures that individuals can engage in activities that suit their fitness level and health status. Here, we provide age-specific exercise guidelines to empower individuals in their journey toward a heart-healthy lifestyle.

Children and Adolescents (Ages 6-17):

Active Play: Encourage children and adolescents to do moderate-to-intense exercise for at least 60 minutes each day. Activities such as running, playing sports, and active games support cardiovascular health and help in weight management.

Strength Training: Include muscle-strengthening activities, like push-ups and squats, at least three times per week. It's essential to focus on proper form and avoid excessive weights, promoting overall strength and fitness.

Limit Sedentary Activities: Minimize screen time and sedentary activities. Encourage breaks from prolonged sitting and promote activities that engage the whole body.

Adults (Ages 18-64)

Aerobic Exercise: Engage in at least 150 minutes of moderate-intensity aerobic exercise or 75 minutes of vigorous-intensity exercise per week. Exercise can be jogging, swimming, cycling, or brisk walking,

Strength Training: Incorporate muscle-strengthening activities on two or more days per week. This can involve weightlifting, bodyweight exercises, or resistance training.

Flexibility and Balance Training: Include flexibility exercises, such as yoga or stretching, and balance training to enhance overall physical fitness.

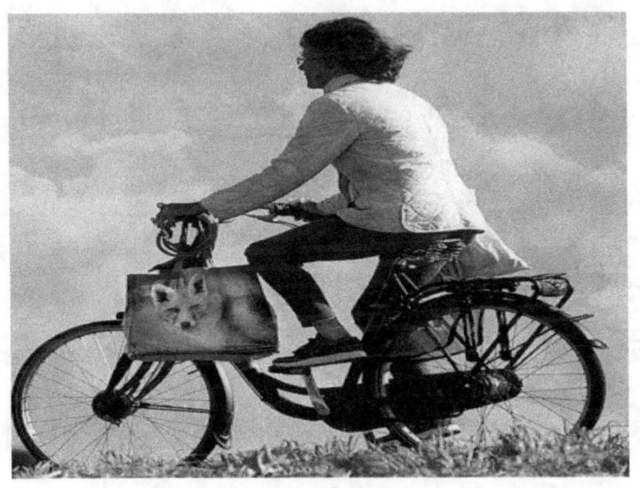

Cycling to work a good exercise technique

Older Adults (Ages 65 and Older)

Moderate-Intensity Activity: Aim for 150 minutes or more a week of moderate-intensity physical activity. Activities like walking, swimming, or dancing can be suitable.

Strength Training: Include strength training activities on two or more days per week. Focus on maintaining muscle mass and bone density, reducing the risk of falls.

Balance and Stability Exercises: Incorporate exercises that enhance balance and stability, reducing the risk of falls. Tai Chi and specific yoga poses can be beneficial.

Before initiating any exercise program, individuals, especially those with pre-existing health conditions such as diabetes, previous history of heart attack, arthritis, and other health conditions, should consult with their healthcare provider to ensure that the chosen activities align with their health status and goals and will not endanger their health further. Tailoring exercise to specific age groups ensures that individuals can enjoy the benefits of physical activity while minimizing the risk of injury or strain. As you embark on this journey of hypertension prevention, by practicing all methods outlined in this handbook, let us celebrate the diversity of fitness and the lifelong commitment to a heart-healthy lifestyle.

Stress Management Techniques

Chronic Stress: In the fast-paced rhythm of modern life, stress has become a ubiquitous companion, affecting not only our mental well-being but also casting shadows on our cardiovascular health. Persistent stress can lead to increased blood pressure. Adopting stress management techniques, including mindfulness, meditation, and relaxation exercises, helps mitigate the physiological impact of stress on the cardiovascular system. This part explores seven effective stress reduction techniques as integral components of hypertension prevention, providing a roadmap to cultivate inner calm and resilience.

1. Mindfulness Meditation: This is a practice that focuses on being present at the moment without judgment. Regular mindfulness sessions, even if brief, can contribute to stress reduction. Techniques such as mindful breathing, body scan, and guided meditation are valuable tools for fostering a sense of calm.

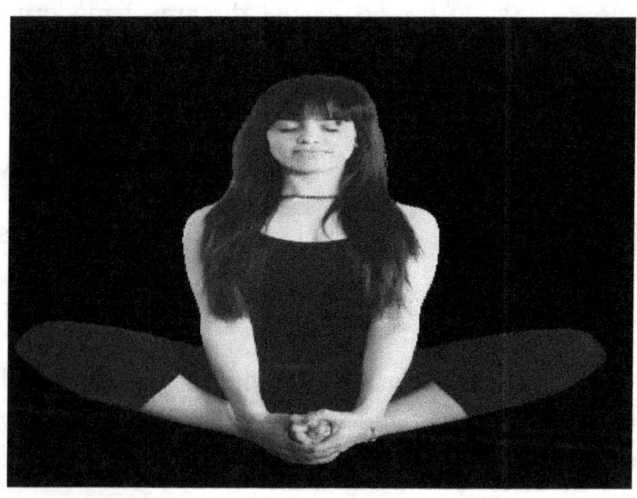

Meditation for mind relaxation

2. Deep Breathing Exercises: Conscious control of our breath can have profound effects on stress levels. Deep breathing exercises, such as diaphragmatic breathing or progressive muscle relaxation, activate the body's relaxation response. Practicing these exercises regularly can contribute to overall stress reduction.

3. Time Management: Effectively managing time and setting realistic goals can reduce the overwhelming feeling of being constantly under pressure. Prioritize tasks, break them into manageable steps, and allow yourself breaks to recharge. Establishing a healthy work-life balance is essential for long-term stress reduction.

4. Social Support: Sharing concerns and experiences with trusted friends, family, or support groups can be a cathartic experience. Social connections provide emotional support, fostering a sense of belonging and resilience against stressors.

5. Relaxation Techniques: Incorporating relaxation techniques into your daily routine can create a buffer against stress. Practices such as progressive muscle relaxation, visualization, or even spending time in nature can promote relaxation and reduce the physiological impact of stress on the body.

6. Hobbies and Leisure Activities: Engaging in activities you enjoy, whether it's reading, gardening, art, or music, serves as a delightful distraction from stressors. Hobbies and leisure activities provide a healthy outlet for creativity and relaxation.

7. Quality sleep: Sleep is a critical component of overall health, and its importance extends to the prevention of hypertension, a significant risk factor for heart disease.

Disturbances in sleep patterns potentially contribute to the development or exacerbation of hypertension.

The appropriate amount of sleep for hypertensive patients, as well as for the general adult population, is typically recommended to be around 7 to 9 hours per night. For hypertensive individuals, adequate and quality sleep is crucial in managing blood pressure and overall cardiovascular health. Chronic sleep deprivation or poor sleep quality has been associated with an increased risk of hypertension and other cardiovascular issues.

Achieving quality sleep involves adopting healthy sleep habits and creating an environment that promotes relaxation.

12 bonus tips for achieving quality sleep to prevent high blood pressure

1. Maintain a Regular Sleep Schedule: Stick to a regular sleep and walk-up time by going to bed and waking up at the same time every day, even on weekends. This aids in the internal clock regulation of the body.

2. Create a Relaxing Bedtime Routine: Develop a pre-sleep routine to signal to your body that it's time to wind down. Activities like taking a warm bath, reading, or practicing relaxation exercises help.

3. Enhance Your Sleep Environment: Keep your bedroom cool, dark, and quiet to create a conducive environment for good sleep. To ensure a restful night's sleep, invest in a comfortable bed, mattress, bedsheets, and pillows.

4. Limit Exposure to Screens Before Bed: The blue light emitted by phones, tablets, and computers can interfere with the production of the sleep hormone melatonin. At least about an hour before going to bed, limit screen time.

5. Monitor Your Diet: Stay away from heavy meals, caffeine or caffeine products, and anything containing nicotine right before bedtime. Their presence in diet can interrupt our normal sleep patterns and make it difficult to sleep.

6. Stay Active During the Day: Retaining regular exercise can help you enjoy a better sleep. Target at least half an hour (30 minutes) of moderate exercise most days of the week; however, stay away from strenuous or intense exercise right before bedtime.

7. Manage Stress: sleep and stress are bidirectional in effect. Practice stress-reducing techniques such as deep breathing, meditation, or mindfulness to help your mind relax before bedtime.

8. Limit Naps: While short naps can be beneficial, long or irregular sleeping during the day can interfere with nighttime sleep. If you must take a nap, take it early in the day and keep it short (20-30 minutes)

9. Assess Your Mattress, bedsheets, and Pillows: Ensure your mattress and pillows are sturdy and comfortable. If your mattress is over 8 years old or if you wake up with aches and pains, it may be time for a new one.

10. Be Mindful of Light Exposure: Exposure to natural light during the day helps regulate your sleep-wake cycle. Spend time outdoors, especially in the morning. At night, keep your bedroom dark to signal to your body that it's time to sleep.

11. Avoid Stimulants Before Bed: Avoid stimulating substances like caffeine and nicotine in the hours leading up to bedtime, as they can interfere with your ability to fall asleep.

12. Seek Professional Help if Needed: If you consistently have difficulty sleeping or experience symptoms of a sleep disorder, such as sleep apnea or insomnia, consult with a healthcare professional for evaluation and guidance.

Adopting these tips and maintaining a consistent sleep routine can contribute significantly to achieving quality sleep and promoting overall well-being.

It's important to note that consistently getting too little or too much sleep can potentially impact blood pressure. Both short sleep duration and excessive sleep have been linked to higher blood pressure levels. Therefore, it's not only about the quantity of sleep but also the quality and consistency.

As we have navigated the intricate relationship between diet, exercise, stress, and hypertension, remember that incorporating these lifestyle techniques into your daily life is not just about preventing high blood pressure; it's an investment in the overall well-being of all organ systems. By cultivating a mindset of calm resilience, and sound and comfortable sleep, you empower yourself on the path to a heart-healthy and harmonious life. Therefore, endeavor to achieve at least seven to nine hours of sleep every day by preventing over and under-sleeping.

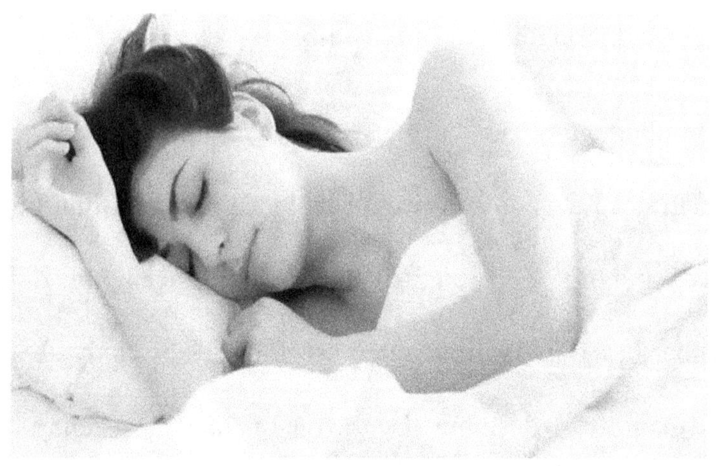

Good Sleep Promotes Good Blood Pressure Control

CHAPTER SIX

Management of Hypertension

Medications play a crucial role in managing hypertension, particularly when lifestyle modifications alone may not be sufficient to control elevated blood pressure. This chapter explores common blood pressure medications, their mechanisms of action, and their role in hypertension prevention.

Secondly hypertension and diabetes act like twin brothers where the presence of one invites the other. Diabetes can quickly lead to hypertension if not properly managed and vice versa. As explained above, the complications of hypertension are dire and include increased ocular pressure or vision impairment through neurovascular destruction.

Other most common complications include heart failure, stroke, kidney impairment, etcetera if not properly managed. Physicians prescribe antihypertensives based on the classification of the high blood pressure, underlying health condition, and the age of the patient. It is therefore recommended to consult a physician or medical practitioner if home blood pressure monitoring is above 130/80mmhg.

Drugs classes and mechanisms of Action

Several classes of medications are employed to lower blood pressure, each targeting different pathways depending on the cause, risk factors, age, and underlying health conditions. Common classes are listed below with their mode of action

Angiotensin-converting enzyme (ACE) and Angiotensin II Receptor Blockers (ARBs):

ACE inhibitors and ARBs work by relaxing blood vessels and reducing the production of angiotensin II—a substance that narrows blood vessels. This opens the blood vessels for smooth blood flow. Examples of **ACE** inhibitors include

Lisinopril (Zestril), Perindopril, Benazepril (Lotensin), Captopril, Enalapril (Vasotec), Fosinopril, and Quinapril.

Example of **ARBs** include Losartan (Cozaar), Olmesartan (Benicar), Telmisartan, Valsartan (Diovan). Candesartan (Atacand), and Irbesartan (Avapro).

Calcium Channel Blockers (CCBs)

Calcium channel blockers (CCBs) are a class of drugs that interfere with the movement of calcium ions into cardiac and smooth muscle cells. They primarily affect L-type calcium channels, which are voltage-gated channels found in the cell membranes of cardiac and smooth muscle cells. The mechanism of action of calcium channel blockers involves blocking these channels, leading to various physiological effects.

In the heart, calcium influx is crucial for the initiation of muscle contraction. By blocking these channels, CCBs reduce the influx of calcium into cardiac muscle cells, leading to a decrease in contractility (negative inotropic effect). This reduces the force and rate of cardiac muscle contraction, making CCBs effective in treating conditions such as hypertension, angina, and certain arrhythmias.

Examples of **CCBs** include nifedipine, amlodipine verapamil, and diltiazem

Diuretics

Diuretics as a class of hypertension medications work by making the body produce more urine to help the body flush out excess salt and water. They are commonly used to treat conditions such as hypertension (high blood pressure), heart failure, kidney disorders, and edema (fluid retention). There are different classes of diuretics, and each class has a slightly different mechanism of action. The three main classes of diuretics are thiazide diuretics, loop diuretics, and potassium-sparing diuretics.

Example of diuretics include hydrochlorothiazide, furosemide, and bumetanide

Beta-Blockers

Beta-blockers, also known as beta-adrenergic blockers exert their effects by blocking the action of catecholamines, such as norepinephrine and epinephrine, at beta-adrenergic receptors. These receptors are found in various tissues throughout the body, including the heart, blood vessels, and certain parts of the central nervous system.

Beta-blockers reduce the heart rate by blocking the action of norepinephrine and epinephrine on beta-1 adrenergic receptors in the heart. They also decrease the force of contraction of the heart muscle, leading to a reduction in the heart's pumping activity.

These effects collectively contribute to a reduction in cardiac output, making beta-blockers useful in conditions such as hypertension, angina, and certain arrhythmias.

Examples of **beta-blockers** include labetalol, metoprolol, propranolol, atenolol, bisoprolol, and carvedilol.

Combination Therapy and Importance of Adherence

In most cases of uncontrolled high blood pressure, a combination of different classes of antihypertensive drugs is prescribed to accomplish normal blood pressure control. Healthcare providers tailor treatment plans based on factors such as age, coexisting health conditions, and potential side effects.

Consistent adherence to prescribed medication regimens is crucial for effective blood pressure control and the prevention of complications. Regular hospital reviews for blood pressure monitoring and adjustment of medications are paramount in controlling hypertension and monitoring. Self-medication and no monitoring are a dangerous road to read. Regular monitoring, coupled with open communication with healthcare providers, helps identify and address potential side effects promptly.

Hypertension in Special Populations

Regular blood pressure monitoring in pediatric populations is crucial for early detection. Monitor blood pressure regularly during pregnancy, especially for the development of gestational hypertension. Early detection is key for appropriate management. Pregnant women should know the signs and symptoms of preeclampsia, a condition characterized by high blood pressure during pregnancy.

Recognize that blood pressure goals may vary for older adults. Individualized targets consider factors such as overall health, functional status, and potential medication interactions.

Routine comprehensive assessments, including diabetes, cognitive function, and frailty, are important for a holistic approach to blood pressure management in older adults.

Individuals with CKD require careful monitoring of blood pressure to prevent further kidney damage. Considerations for medication choice and dosages are critical in individuals with CKD to manage blood pressure effectively.

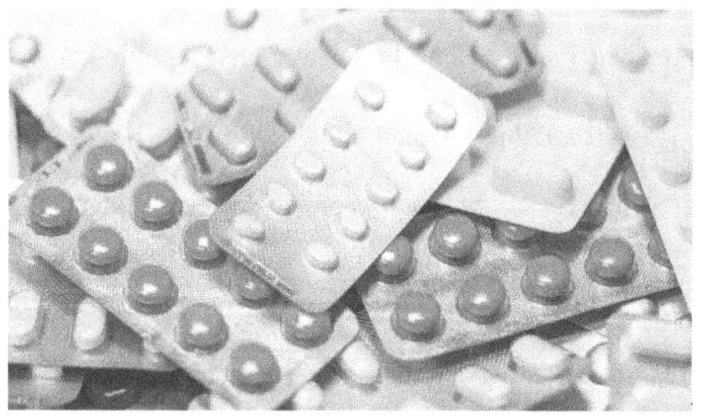

CHAPTER SEVEN

Complications of hypertension

Diabetes and Hypertension: Diabetes and hypertension often coexist, creating a bidirectional relationship. Controlling blood pressure in individuals with diabetes is crucial for preventing cardiovascular complications.

Lifestyle modifications, including a heart-healthy diet, regular physical activity, and glucose control, are foundational in managing both conditions.

Hypertension and Cardiovascular Disease: Hypertension is a major risk factor for atherosclerosis and cardiovascular diseases. Managing blood pressure is essential for preventing heart attacks and strokes

A comprehensive approach to risk reduction involves addressing modifiable factors, including blood pressure, cholesterol levels, and lifestyle choices.

Cardiovascular Complications:

Heart Failure: Hypertension can strain the heart over time, leading to heart failure. Timely blood pressure control helps reduce the risk of heart failure.

Stroke: Hypertension is a leading cause of stroke, contributing to the formation of blood clots or the rupture of blood vessels in the brain. Blood pressure control is paramount in stroke prevention.

Dementia: Untreated hypertension can increase the risk of vascular dementia due to reduced blood flow to the brain. Managing blood pressure supports cognitive health.

High Blood Pressure and Renal Complications: Hypertension is a primary cause of CKD. Strict blood pressure control is essential in preventing the progression of kidney damage. Persistent uncontrolled hypertension can lead to End-Stage Renal Disease (ESRD), necessitating dialysis or transplantation. Aggressive blood pressure management is crucial in delaying or preventing ESRD.

Hypertension and Eye Complications:

Retinopathy: Hypertension contributes to retinal damage, leading to hypertensive retinopathy. Blood pressure control is vital in preventing vision-related complications.

Severe hypertensive retinopathy can lead to vision impairment or loss, emphasizing the importance of timely blood pressure management.

Conclusion

From the knowledge we have gained from this book, we can all make conclusions from the introductory story of Madam Caroline.

The first thing noted from her social history is that she could be genetically exposed because her mother died of a heart attack. Secondly, she grew up in an environment where she had to consume a lot of iodized salt which predisposed her to thyroid diseases-main reason for her poorly controlled blood pressure.

She also had to endure a lot of stress at work coupled with poor dietary habits such as late supper with no physical activity.

Most of these risk factors in Madam Caroline were directly under her control because when she was counseled on lifestyle modifications coupled with proper treatment of the ensuing hyperthyroidism, her blood pressure was put under her control and she regained her heart health.

Human survival is dependent on our ability to decipher between good and bad and this book has empowered us on the journey to heart health. If you master the strategies elaborated in this book and practice them, you shall be in charge of your heart and take possession of your health.

Enjoy your heart-healthy journey

Here We Are: Normal Blood Pressure Maintained